THE G-JO INSTITUTE "SELF-HEALTH" PROGRAM FOR TREATING YOUR OWN ARTHRITIS

published by The G-Jo Institute

Arthritis—the dread crippler that affects women five times more frequently than men—seems to be caused, in part, by a combination of imbalanced or incomplete nutrition plus harsh, unresolved emotional distress. It is primarily a chronic joint disability that includes nearly 100 different symptoms. "Arthritis" is actually a catch-all or umbrella term that includes *osteoarthritis, rheumatoid arthritis, bursitis, rheumatism, gout, menopausal arthritis, etc.*

Arthritis has been called "The Resentment Disease," "The Hidden Anger Disease," "The Woman's Crippler," etc. And while it is primarily a disorder of the joints, it may affect bones, ligaments, tendons and even organs, as well. Arthritic symptoms usually begin manifesting themselves before the age of forty. Arthritis has been treated medically by numerous substances; and while some medical therapies have been temporarily effective, most have proven themselves eventually useless or even harmful. Several common medications are frequently used to relieve arthritis—aspirin, gold, cortisone and "The Pill" (oral contraceptive)—all of which have potentially harmful side-effects.

If you are planning on reversing arthritis naturally—that is, healing yourself without taking further drugs or harsh medications—please discuss this course of action first with your doctor. Then withdraw from any present medication gradually, not suddenly, especially if you have been taking medication for a long time.

All disease creates inconvenience. The greater the disease, the greater its inconvenience. Arthritis creates substantial inconvenience if you are going to reverse (heal) your disease as completely as possible. You should be aware of this, because your arthritis has taken many years to "accumulate" and it will take some time to reverse itself. So please allow yourself to be patient with this program of self-health methods and techniques.

Arthritis is often associated with excessively low blood pH (too acid. . . a hyperacid system). Certain "extreme" foods—especially those which create or continue this state of hyperacidity—appear to "leach out" needed nutrients from the system, so you must avoid those foods as much as possible (details below). But proper eating is not enough to totally reverse arthritis, because it did not begin with food—arthritis is rooted in the emotions. Therefore, you'll have to use other therapies—methods which deal with the emotions as well as the pain of arthritis—in conjunction with any dietary tactics.

There are nine important categories in The G-Jo Institute self-health program for healing your own arthritis. The information in each category plays a vital part in creating a "whole-person" or *holistic* approach for healing yourself. Please read this entire program before beginning any techniques or methods described herein. The nine categories are:

1. **good preventative and/or therapeutic foods**
2. **common excesses, abuses or irritants**
3. **preventative and/or therapeutic vitamins**
4. **preventative and/or therapeutic minerals and other supplements**
5. **other common needs and deficiencies of arthritis sufferers**
6. **important "external" therapies (e.g., exercise, etc.)**
7. **preventative and/or other therapeutic herbs or other "natural medicines"**
8. **meditation plus specific prayers and visualizations**
9. **important "acupressure" (acupuncture without needles) methods and techniques**

Illness cannot be divided between body and mind, for body and mind are actually one and the same. "Mind" extends from—and is thus linked to—the various organs and the biochemicals they produce. And the "bodymind," according to many holistically-oriented healers, is a manifestation of the spiritual part of the human being—the part sometimes called the "soul."

Ultimately, it is said, *all* disease represents spiritual imbalance within the sufferer, so no complete healing is possible unless and until *spiritual* well-being is restored. It is our experience that some kind of spiritual practice greatly aids the process of healing.

There are at least 12 major organs within your body and each of these directly or indirectly controls one or more mental/emotional functions, according to holistic healers from the East. This unusual idea—that organs are "in charge" of emotions and various mental activities—is now becoming more widely accepted even in traditional medical circles. In short, one's emotional state appears to be directly related to his electro-chemical balance. When this mixture is is too "rich" in one biochemical—say, insulin (a product of the liver interacting with the spleen, pancreas and other digestive organs)—predictable emotional responses nearly always occur (in this case anger, depression and/or hostility).

Furthermore, an excess of one or more biochemicals must also produce a deficiency in others. Thus, the effects of imbalance within your system are two-sided and create many complicated problems. Until better electro-chemical balance is restored, these problems will continue to cause your arthritis to plague you.

Each food, thought and activity is believed to have an immediate result on the electro-chemical mixture. The goal of this natural self-health program is to restore proper electro-chemical balance—and to help you maintain it as completely as possible—through regular therapeutic practices and avoidances. When balance is restored, your arthritis will diminish.

Before starting this program, it is important for you to think about—and accept—several important facts about your disease:

1. **something—and often many things—in your lifestyle are unhealthy and contributing to your illness**

2. **you are ill and suffering, not just from arthritis, but from emotional and spiritual imbalance, as well**

3. **to become well and reverse your disease, you must first WANT to get well . . . the intention to heal yourself is as important as any therapy or technique; without that intention to get well, you can never enjoy prime health and well-being!**

4. **while many of these techniques are surprisingly easy, all of them have helped others heal themselves of arthritis; but you must allow yourself enough time for the techniques to show substantial effects . . . and while you may notice some benefits almost immediately, solid results could take a month or longer to appear.**

THE EMOTIONS WHICH ARE CONNECTED TO ARTHRITIS: Arthritis is best characterized by *emotional inflexibility* and a *low "adaptability factor."* Female arthritis sufferers often hold strong "romantic" illusions—such as fairy tale notions or impossibly high ideals—about what life "should be." At the core of this fantasy is usually found the sufferer's attitude about male-female relationships and her reaction to it—nearly always one of *resentment.* The greater a woman resents her (real or imagined) role as a female, the greater her potential of suffering from arthritis. Male arthritis sufferers often carry hidden anger and resentment directed towards employers or superiors in business or work. Rheumatoid arthritis is often suffered by someone who hides resentment and hostility by "putting on a good face." Osteoarthrititis sufferers are often unusually *fearful.* Gout—which is generally triggered by a rich, fatty diet—may be rooted in hidden fears of *deprivation* and *starvation* (a common emotional symptom of obesity, too). Other forms of arthritis have their own, special emotional wellsprings, as well.

While it is possible to intellectually understand that these emotions may exist within you, becoming *fully* aware of their influence is far more difficult. The pain and suffering from your arthritis may actually be serving the purpose of *protecting* you from having to directly confront those hard-to-handle feelings. But until you recognize that your unvented emotions and feelings *are* the roots of your illness, the most you can expect is temporary relief from suffering.

Though arthritis affects the entire bodymind, there are three major organs which are primarily responsible for your state of arthritic suffering: the *lungs . . .* the *kidneys . . .*and the *liver.* Only by restoring these organs to a better state of balance and functioning can arthritis be reversed and healed. Left unchecked and uncontrolled, however, the arthritic man or woman may expect to suffer from at least several of these common symptoms:

- **gall bladder problems**
- **low or erratic blood pressure**
- **deformed hands, feet**
- **anemia**
- **colitis**
- **constipation**
- **dry skin, mucous membranes, etc.**
- **bronchitis and night cough**
- **wry neck**
- **craving for acids, acidy foods**
- **acute allergic reactions**
- **cataracts or other eye problems**
- **painful toes and fingers**

nearly constant pain
edema in the ankles
emotional distress
bone spurs
tendency to form kidney stones
frequent leg cramps
joint stiffness
arteriosclerosis, etc.

As you see, whatever small inconvenience you may experience in changing your diet and "healthstyle" will be greatly rewarded by reducing—even avoiding—the above symptoms (most of which will be *very* inconvenient . . . and unpleasant).

There are well over 100 foods, supplements, techniques and methods which have been successfully used to control and reverse arthritis. Please read the following pages staying open intuitively to any foods, vitamins, minerals, herbs or methods that "feel right," seem "good for me," "sound tasty," etc. You already have a subtle knowledge of what is right for you—allowing this to "bloom" will be a most important tool in your job of healing yourself. First try those foods or methods that are most appealing. Use several—even many—for it doesn't matter *what* remedies help you—only that they do work to bring relief and stimulate self-healing.

FOODS WHICH OFTEN HELP RELIEVE AND REVERSE ARTHRITIS (try to build your diet around these . . . most important are in bold face type):

grapefruit (including the white membrane)
yoghurt
buttermilk
strawberries
sour apples
kelp (a sea vegetable)
millet
brown rice
sesame seeds or tahini
sunflower seeds
wheat bran
tofu (bean curd)
agar-agar
asparagus
broccoli
rutabagas
pumpkin seeds
raw goat's milk
green, leafy vegetables
red beets
wheat grass (sprouted wheat seeds)
watercress
potatoes (juice of raw potatoes)
yams
celery
parsley
garbanzos
sauerkraut (be careful of salt)
rice bran
pectin (e.g., "Certo")
parsnips
squash
lettuce

peas	chard
carrots	cauliflower
endive	oatmeal
sour cherries	bananas
pineapple	wheat germ
most beans (dried)	avacados
pecans	**alfalfa, especially sprouted**
fresh tomato juice	most bean sprouts
turnips	**string beans**

We strongly recommend a vegetarian diet, with the main emphasis on fresh fruits and vegetables picked within 50 miles of home. It is important to remember that *food, itself, does not cure—it only stimulates the bodymind, through the organs, to heal itself.* For this reason, moderation is extremely important in taking food and drink. Even the "best" foods taken in excess can create chaos in the bodymind. Chewing for a long time—because of its effect on the liver, a main organ for controlling one's sensitivity to pain—is almost as important as the food itself. In short, *chew small bites of "right" foods for a long time (up to 100 times).*

We believe *any* meat or slaughtered product is unhealthy because when a creature is slaughtered, its terror chemicals infect the meat. Aside from being unnecessary and inhumane, the end product of the slaughtered creature's terror hormones and biochemicals finds its way into the ultimate consumer. This creates and fuels a high level of stress, fear and tension within the consumer—a condition which a sufferer from arthritis is trying to avoid.

Arthritis sufferers should have at least one meal daily consisting of raw vegetables, either whole or in the form of fresh juice. An interesting way to serve raw vegetables—even if you hate raw foods—is as a "blended salad." The best way to prepare a blended salad is to use a food processor and simply chop any fresh, local vegetables for a few moments, until some juice is seen on the bottom of the processor. Add a few drops of fresh lemon juice and cayenne (red pepper) for "snap" and enjoy! Raw horseradish, too, can be a healthful addition. But please avoid salt—or, if you must use it, try a sea salt/vegetable combination available from your local whole- or health-food store.

Your cooked vegetables should be *steamed*, rather than fried, boiled or baked, etc. Steamed foods benefit the liver most, the organ which is primarily responsible for controlling your tolerance or sensitivity to pain. A hyperactive liver—which often reveals its condition through *anger, hostility, inward-turned aggressive emotions, loud voice, flatulence, bowel disorders, frequent cursing (either verbalized or silently, in your own mind),* etc.—practically guarantees that you will suffer more pain than someone whose liver is in better balance.

Raw fruit juices, too, are recommended—in moderation. We suggest you use these as replacements for coffee, soft drinks (especially colas), tea, chocolate-based or alcoholic beverages. Nearly any raw fruit or vegetable juice—except *cabbage* and sweet citrus, such as *orange* or *tangerine*—has at least neutral and usually beneficial or therapeutic qualities. But caffeinated or sugary beverages have quite the reverse effect and seem to stimulate pain.

COMMON EXCESSES, ABUSES OR IRRITANTS THAT TRIGGER ARTHRITIC SYMPTOMS: There are a number of foods and other irritants that arthritis sufferers need to avoid as much as possible. The most important dietary avoidances include:

sugar or sugary foods and drinks	most seafoods, especially herring, anchovies, sardines and shellfish
slaughtered animal products, including organ meats, chicken, turkey, cold cuts or any other meat products	eggs sweet citrus fruits macaroni and spaghetti eggplant white bread, other refined wheat products
salt	
red or green peppers	paprika

most dairy products, especially milk, ice cream, whipped cream and any pasteurized product.

Since the above list includes most of the staples of today's "normal" American diet, it is not difficult to understand why arthritis is such a widespread disorder.

This is not to say that these foods necessarily *cause* arthritis—but they do trigger extreme emotional states by throwing the body-mind into electro-chemical imbalance. When this occurs for a long period of time—months or years—negative emotions become fixed, perceptions are altered and one's viewpoint becomes restricted.

Besides abusive foods and drinks, there are a number of other excesses, health disorders and abuses which are intimately related to arthritis and its suffering:

- **smoking** (especially harmful to women)
- malnutrition—even many overweight people suffer from malnutrition, too
- physical stress
- emotional tension
- **"hidden" food allergies**
- obesity (being more than 10% above ideal body weight)
- alkalosis—being too alklaine in the stomach (caused by too many *acidy* foods—such as sugar—strangely enough)
- injuries and other physical traumas

This list is not necessarily complete as to the causes, excesses or abuses which trigger arthritis and the emotions that seem to lead to it. But nearly all the above are proven arthritis-linked abuses that can be curtailed, eliminated or eased without great difficulty.

Hidden food allergies, however, are another problem. Everyone has them—often to important staples of their diets which do not appear on the list of "wrong" foods. As a rule of thumb, generally those foods which we crave and would miss the most are the most highly suspect. Any food taken to excess has the possibility of causing an "addiction"—which is closely related to food allergy—although there are other methods for locating hidden food allergens, methods which are far more dependable.

The bodymind reveals its allergies in many ways. One of the most apparent is in the change of the *pulse rate.* If your pulse rises more than five percent following a meal, the chances are high that you've consumed something that you're allergic to. A more complete description of this method for finding your own hidden food allergies is discussed in Dr. Arthur Coca's *The Pulse Test: Easy Allergy Detection* (Arc Books, Arco Publishing Co., NY).

The bodymind already contains *everything* it needs to heal even the most grievous of illnesses. *Why* it fails to do so without our conscious, voluntary efforts is a complex question to answer and ultimately leads into the realm of spirituality, purpose for being alive and other esoteric questions.

But unless you are well-trained in the field of holistic therapy, these "questions without easy answers" may be temporarily set aside until other, more practical areas of healing are first explored. For example, while food and nutrition may not actually heal the bodymind, no true well-being is possible until a big, first step—that of becoming food-conscious—is taken. Being food-conscious means being aware of the emotional/mental effects (as well as the physiological effects, of course) that food has on our bodyminds. This is no easy task. It usually means first a period of self-deprivation to "cleanse" the system of its most gross "toxins." These toxins—which are actually hormonal and energy imbalances that manifest themselves as "organ warps" (malfunctions)—may take many years to fully purge (if ever), but a vast majority of them are released in the first weeks or months of a dietary change—especially if one becomes a vegetarian in the beginning.

On the other hand, however, simply eating the "right" foods without taking into consideration many of the other factors associated, not only with arthritis, but with *any* illness can only bring limited, temporary success. And trying to cure illness exclusively through dietary controls holds an added threat—that of becoming "food proud" or intolerant about any diet other than one's own.

PREVENTATIVE AND/OR THERAPEUTIC VITAMINS: Arthritis creates/is created by *deficiencies* as well as excesses and other abuses. One of the most important deficiencies is a *lack of certain vitamins.* Vitamins appear to be created within the organs—they do not need to be "extracted" (in fact, it is possible they *cannot* be extracted) from food. Food appears to *stimulate* the organs to produce their respective vitamins. But this stimulation can occur from other sources, as well. Sunshine, for instance, produces vitamin D (ergosterol) when it irradiates the skin. And vitamin B_{12}—the vitamin vegetarians try to find in sources other than meat—is produced in the large intestine (colon), stimulated in such unusual ways as walking barefoot in grass which still holds early morning dew for as little as 10 minutes a day!

Nutritional deficiencies may be temporarily remedied by taking oral supplements to provide the following vitamins (as well as mineral and other nutritional needs). However, vitamin pills should be taken only for a limited amount of time, in our opinion—perhaps as long as a year—and used in conjunction with the other methods described in this program. *There is no single path to reversing arthritis—it must be a holistic effort.* And while vitamin pills may be catalysts that trigger reversal, rejuvenation and healing of illness, so may they also create a dependency or "vitamin addiction."

The following vitamins have proven themselves useful in self-treatment of arthritis:

B complex
extra B_2 (riboflavin)
extra B_3 (niacin)
extra B_5 (pantothenic acid)
extra B_6 (pyridoxine)
extra B_{12} (cobalamin)
vitamin A
vitamin C —up to 5 gm. daily
vitamin D
vitamin E
vitamin P (bioflavinoids)

Since each person is unique, it is difficult to suggest ideal amounts of each vitamin to take. A good suggestion is to begin by taking slightly more than is recommended on the bottle for several days, then reducing it to the suggested level on the label. If you notice no beneficial effects, add more—gradually. But if you notice any negative effects, you must test to see which of the supplements is causing the problem. For this reason, we suggest you use separate pills for each vitamin, rather than taking a heavy multiple vitamin and mineral pill. First add those vitamins which are in bold-face type. Please remember: *Fresh foods grown locally are your best source of vitamins and other nutritional needs.*

Common symptoms of excessive vitamin intake (hypervitaminosis) may include nausea, diarrhea, rashes, etc. Such problems occur most frequently with excesses of niacin, vitamin A and vitamin D. Not only excess nutrients, but even reputedly beneficial foods—such as "harmless" parsley—can be the source of unpleasant health problems when consumed to excess. *More is better than less* and *sooner is better than later* apply only to money and success, not arthritis. Fast "cures" for diseases that have taken a long time to accumulate are highly suspect and appear to be contradictory to the laws of nature.

PREVENTATIVE AND/OR THERAPEUTIC MINERALS AND OTHER SUPPLEMENTS: Not only vitamins, but certain minerals and elements are depleted as arthritis "blooms." Even the body-mind manufactures these—through a process called "biological transmutation" (described more completely in *Biological Transmutations*, by Dr. L. Kervran, Swan House Publishing Co., Brooklyn, NY)—trom a wide variety of sources when in good health. The following supplements will help relieve the mineral deficiencies suffered by arthritics:

dolomite (provides necessary magnesium and calcium—an arthritic needs up to 500 mg daily of each mineral)
hydrogen
potassium
bromelain (pineapple enzyme)
hydrochloric acid (HCL)
sodium (through vegetables and herbs, not table salt)
iodine
sulpher
zinc

Here, too—as with vitamins—fresh fruits and vegetables are your best source of most minerals (dolomite being the exception).

Two easy "folk" remedies for easing arthritis also help provide necessary minerals and elements. The first is to mix *epsom salts and cream of tartar in a glass of water* (a small amount of each, taken twice daily). The second—wearing a *copper bracelet or anklet*—appears to have an electrolytic balancing effect on arthritis sufferers' systems. However, copper is a highly toxic and active metal, and non-arthritic people should generally avoid wearing this metal. It is easily absorbed through the skin and may actually create pain in the joints of otherwise healthy people.

OTHER COMMON NEEDS AND DEFICIENCIES OF ARTHRITIS SUFFERERS: There are several other common deficiencies found in arthritis patients. Their remedies will be included in the following section. Several of these deficiencies are:

low blood oxygen levels
lack of regular exercise
a method for expressing hidden emotions that is both direct as well as non-destructive

IMPORTANT "EXTERNAL" THERAPIES: As hidden emotions —unresolved emotions—build, their "results" tend to lodge themselves in the joints of the body(mind). That is a capsule view of arthritis. Disperse these results and arthritis is being reversed. There are a number of ways of helping this process, aside from the previously mentioned dietary controls. The most important of these conscious, voluntary therapies are:

moderate exercise
breath controls
acupressure (separate section for this technique)
self-psychotherapy
prayer and meditation (separate section for these techniques)

The exercise program we recommend is based on *stretching and movement*. We suggest avoiding harsh, violent exercise or sports and focusing, instead, on a kind of free-form, unstructured dancing—done preferrably outside in the sunlight—until a light sheen of perspiration forms across the brow and shoulders. Ideally, this "slow dance" should be done to the beat of Gregorian chants or other church-like music. In fact, the slower the movements, the better. As you move, grace is less important than stretching—especially stretching the extremities—and each muscle should get some benefits of the movement. Doing this for just a few minutes a day is often enough exercise to be energising and invigorating. For many arthritis sufferers, freedom from pain is measured in minutes, not hours, and slow dance will often bring long spans of "relief time"—especially when combined with other parts of this self-health program.

For many sufferers, *hatha yoga* and its many postures and poses has brought relief. If you follow the path of yoga, however, please be sure to allow yourself enough rest time between poses for the full benefits of this activity to occur. With yoga, it is the stretching which allows certain harmful biochemicals to be released, but it is the resting which allows them to be purged into the excretory system. You only need to hold the pose long enough to feel a sense of tiredness—that is the indication these biochemicals have been released. Holding a pose longer than that, or "competing"—either against yourself or someone in a yoga class to see who can hold a difficult pose the longest—is totally contrary to the nature and purpose of this otherwise useful technique.

A most useful exercise is *walking* (usually 300—400 lively steps a day is enough, especially if you are a vegetarian). *Bicycling* and *swimming* are other very beneficial moderate exercises, too. In all forms of exercise, we believe that it is the *quality*—not the quantity—of the exercise that counts. That all parts of the system, especially the joints of the extremities, receive some flexion is more important than for a few parts to receive strenuous activity while others lie dormant; try to shake your wrists, fingers and ankles no matter what kind of exercise you do. Even cracking your knuckles—if you suffer from regular pain there—is a good form of stretching and flexion. And with a little forethought, nearly any activity you do can be made into some beneficial kind of exercise or therapy. All it takes is desire and a bit of imagination.

Learning to directly—but *non-destructively*—confront important sources of emotional irritants that trigger arthritis is more difficult than exercising or controlling your diet. But until you do find a way to deal with these hidden or stashed emotions, any other therapy is only going to have limited results. If you are an arthritic woman, this may mean confronting a husband, son and/or father. If you are an arthritic man, it may well mean confronting an employer. In either case, it raises a very uncomfortable spectre—having that person either be very hurt or even say back to you: "if you don't like it here, get out!" Whether real or imagined, if you can identify with this fear, you'll need some "strong medicine"—in the form of self-psychotherapy—to get past this important hurdle.

There are two problems: much or most of the harsh emotions you feel are really *not* justified, but simply misunderstandings and misconceptions on your part, fed and fueled by the food you eat and the lifestyle you live; but if they *are* justified reactions to important people in your life, you are probably dealing with insensitive types who wouldn't understand what you're talking about.

We suggest *keeping a daily journal*. If you find that too hard or inconvenient, take a few minutes each day to *talk to a wall.* Not just *think* to a wall, but actually verbalize your thoughts and feelings openly, as best as possible, to your "wailing wall." If you have a guru or spiritual master (such as Jesus), it may help greatly to have His picture placed in front of you to look at. If not, perhaps a pretty painting or photograph—even just a spot to meditate upon.

Openly verbalizing and/or writing your grievances, complaints and such is an excellent safety valve for easing the pressures that drive harsh emotions deeper within, but which only express themselves later as pain and suffering. Keeping a daily journal stimulates important insights and self-revelations plus provides you a permanent, ongoing record of your exciting voyage toward self-health and well-being. In every case of arthritis, it is the sufferer's attitude—real or imagined—that is at the root of the problem. Reviewing your daily record will soon show you where the problems lie—and often highlight their solutions.

As mentioned earlier, the lungs—in conjunction with the liver and the kidneys—appear to play an important part in the process of arthritis. In fact, according to many healers throughout history, the lungs play a rich part in the creation, maintenance and destruction of most diseases. Of all the major organs, the lungs are the most easily "reached" for self-therapy. And the therapy, itself, is very simple: *deep, controlled breathing done in series several times a day!* At the most, it takes one or two minutes and may be done anywhere and nearly any time.

Any kind of deep breathing exercise will be helpful, as long as you take at least ten deep breaths—filling your lungs to capacity—then exhale as deeply as you can. But there are specific ways of breathing deeply which magnify this technique's effectiveness.

One excellent method of deep breathing—one that has been practiced by disciples of hatha yogis for many centuries—consists simply of a 2-1-2-1 cycle. This means that for every two counts of inhaled or exhaled breath you take, you hold it for one (at the "top" and "bottom" of the cycle). For example: Begin your breathing cycle by totally emptying your lungs; then gradually draw in a long breath—drawing it in from as low in your abdomen as you can through your nostrils—for, say, a count of ten. Then hold your breath for a count of five . . . exhale on a measured, gradual basis for another ten count . . . and sit quietly with your lungs emptied for another five count. Do this in a series of ten and do it at least twice daily.

Within several weeks of consciously controlling your breath in this manner, you'll actually find yourself breathing more deeply and regularly . . . feeling calmer and less prone to anger . . . and more able to keep centered in previously emotion-filled situations.

Several variations on that theme are to read as much of a paragraph of a newspaper as you can on your out-breath (and, of course, trying to empty your lungs as completely as possible in the process). Your in-breath should be as deep and slow as you can manage.

Another variation is the *cleansing*—or hyperventilating—breath cycle. This is simply rapid, deep breathing (most people can't reach a count of ten without feeling very lightheaded at first) done several times a day. Still another method involves closing one side of the nostril with a thumb or finger on the in-breath, then opening that side and closing the other on the out-breath. It requires more concentration and control to avoid rushing or panicking in the process. But the normal deep, slow breathing as first described is quite adequate for greatly adding to your other self-

-health efforts and techniques and their benefits.

The biggest difficulty is retraining yourself to breathe. Very few people actually take more than very shallow breaths, except under rare circumstances—yawning, smoking a cigarette or after intense physical activity, for instance—and remembering to practice your deep breathing exercises in the beginning of your self-health program is essential. However, after you make several days of conscious effort, it will begin becoming a normal activity and soon become a regular part of your breathing cycle.

There are several other important external therapies which have been beneficial to many arthritis sufferers. *Oil balms and massages* have long been a favorite of self-healthers for speedy, effective relief. Of the various oils often recommended, three—*olive, peanut and castor oils*—appear most frequently in natural healing "prescriptions." Their use is simple enough: Just rub the selected oil into the sore areas, especially the most painful joints. However, when using castor oil, it is best to avoid inflamed areas.

While these oils may be used cold (at room temperature), when the oily area is covered with a layer of cloth and a heating pad to make a *radiant oil treatment*, the effectiveness is greatly increased. The greater the arthritic suffering, the longer these radiant oil packs should stay in place—perhaps up to several hours, in some cases. They are best done during a time of relaxation—say, just before an afternoon nap or at bedtime.

Another useful way to apply heat for easing arthritic suffering is to take a long, hot bath—then quickly follow that with a brief, cold shower. And since warmth seems so important in the treatment of arthritis, try *sleeping in a sleeping bag* to maintain a uniform sense of warmth throughout the night.

Sunlight has a beneficial effect, too. If possible, expose your face to sunlight for at least 15 minutes daily—perhaps while doing your slow dancing routine out-of-doors—and keep your eyes open. This is a very effective way for accelerating healing since it has a profound effect on the liver. Do not look directly into the sun, but look as near to it as possible until discomfort occurs, then look slightly away.

The use of *poultices*—packs of crushed herbs or other vegetable substances—is an art that is returning to popularity after being mostly ignored by Americans for many decades. The most common way to make a poultice is to crush an herbal root or complete plant—*comfrey* is one of the best for arthritic suffering (see section below)—and either place this mash directly on the skin or (more commonly) on a light cotton cloth (perhaps a piece of bedsheet) and wrap the pack with another piece of cloth. Let it stay in place for as long as possible. Many different plants and herbs have been used for poultices—even *common grass!*—so don't be afraid to experiment. It is said by many natural healers that the nearer to one's home the therapeutic plant or herb grows, the more beneficial it is.

PREVENTATIVE AND/OR THERAPEUTIC HERBS AND OTHER NATURAL "MEDICINES": Self-healthing your way out of the arthritis cycle may begin with changes in diet, but there is more to healing than adding "good" foods and subtracting "bad" ones. Another important aspect in healing your own arthritis is the use of herbs and medicinal spices.

Like good food and nutritional supplements, herbal remedies appear to stimulate the appropriate organs into self-correcting and -balancing (healing) activities. There are literally hundreds of thousands of medicinal plants—some Oriental healers say *every* plant or flower has a medicinal value—and there are certainly hundreds of such plants that are specifically beneficial for arthritis sufferers.

Unless otherwise specified, these herbs and spices should be taken as *teas* or *infusions* and consumed several times a day, after being steeped for a minimum of 15 minutes. Don't throw any herbal tea away—instead, drink it cool, at room temperature. Use it instead of water, at least in the beginning. If you find there are several of these herbal teas you like, mix them. The highest and most experienced herbalists usually suggest using blends of three, four or even five teas for chronic problems. Again, used alone and without other therapeutic practices, herbal therapy usually takes many months for satisfying results to occur. But when used in conjunction with other remedies and avoidances, they are imporant supplements to speed along your self-health program. Here are some of the most popular herbs for treating arthritis:

- ginseng (men only)
- black cohosh
- sarsaparilla
- birch leaves
- skullcap
- juniper berries
- ginger (especially fresh root)
- mistletoe

yucca	poke berries
valerian (use cautiously)	sassafras
buckthorn bark	fenugreek
dandelion	peach tree leaves (especially gout)
goldenseal	slippery elm
peppermint	burdock
ragwort	yarrow
mountain flax	comfrey
chaparral	rosemary
nettles	sage

There are a number of other edibles—spices, cooking aids and such—which are very useful in relieving and reversing arthritis. These should be used in moderation, of course—somewhere between the small dosages of herbs, usually, and the larger servings of staples. They include:

garlic	sea water (2-3 tbsp. daily)
onions	brewer's yeast (careful of allergy)
lecithin	chives
apple cider vinegar (plus water, as a "cocktail")	**olive oil** (both for cooking and with salads)
capsicum (cayenne)	**raw** cream (if you can find it)

MEDITATION PLUS SPECIFIC PRAYERS OR VISUALIZATIONS: Prayerful meditation is a technique which could fill several books on its own, and it involves three, specific steps for its greatest effectiveness to be realized:

1. prayer
2. meditation
3. visualization

The prayer is to God or Universal Spirit (or whatever "higher" Force you may believe exists within/outside of yourself), urging It to reveal to you, in your meditation (or in whatever fashion It chooses), the source and reason for the hostile, aggressive feelings you may sense you have at the root of your illness. In your prayer, it is important to ask for help in revealing to yourself your *own* part in the process. Ask to have the source—the deep, hidden source—of your anger revealed . . . and to be presented with ways for dealing with anger in the highest, best method for all concerned. Pray for help in recognizing that it is *your* anger, hostility and resentment, caused only by you and allowed into your bodymind *only* with your permission . . .

Upon completing your prayer, become meditative. Don't try to "force" meditation—meditation is a *passive* technique, not active, and it simply means listening *without judgement* to what's going on in your mind. Try to relax as much as possible—sit comfortably or lie down. Don't be concerned if you can't seem to stay focused and attentive to all the mental activity. It's OK—the relaxation is the most important part of this step.

Then, when it feels right, take a positive step out of the meditative state by beginning to visualize the breaking up and dispersing of the "stone" that binds your joints and makes them painful to move. Visualize your joints—especially the most tender and painful ones—as being "cemented" tightly together, but that a gentle, warm solvent is starting to flow in your system to dissolve that cement. In their place, feel love, light, warmth and relaxation. Then send that same love, light and warmth outward, from your heart, toward those closest to you—especially those most directly "responsible" for your arthritis. As you "broadcast" this loving warmth, feel fresh, vital tissue replacing the old, cemented tissue and boney areas . . .

This prayerful meditation is best done during two specific times —*when you have the least time to do it* (e.g., when you're rushed or under stress—the times your anger and hostility is most likely to be at the forefront of your mood); and, of course, at bedtime. Another good time for performing this technique (which only takes a few minutes, with practice) is just before arising. If possible, awaken 15 minutes earlier than usual. But if you have to rush through the process—don't. It's better to arise relaxed than to feel tense and hurried just to meditate. It can't be done, in fact.

As with breathing techniques, there are many possible variations. One good method involves relaxing the area above, between and below the eyes (liver- and kidney-related areas), and along the sides of the mouth (lung-related). Then focus relaxation to the liver area (just below the right breast, above the bottom of the rib cage), trying to calm and balance it as much as possible. Then focus on the lungs, trying to become aware of any hostility and angry words shrinking tighter and tighter into a little ball floating in the middle of your lungs and, when small enough, being exhaled into the universe for purification (you may actually have coughing spasms in the beginning of this practice). Then move your focus to the lower middle back—the kidney area—and try to feel your kidneys "unkink" and ease as you send radiant warmth and light to them . . .

The variations are endless. And if you already have a meditative or self-relaxation technique, these are good ways to expand it. But whatever method you use, always make sure that you close (or awaken yourself) with suggestion that you forgive yourself, forgive those who are linked to your arthritis, and feel love for all—especi*ally for yourself!*

IMPORTANT "ACUPRESSURE" (acupuncture without needles) METHODS AND TECHNIQUES: Acupressure is an ancient Oriental self-health art that relies on fingertip pressure to stimulate the body's tiny therapy points. There are more than 1200 of these pinhead-sized points, of which 116 are highly pressure-responsive. This technique is one of the most effective known remedies for both relieving pain quickly (usually within 10 or 15 *seconds!*) and helping to stimulate the bodymind's own self-healing mechanisms.

These techniques are more fully described in our publication number 1001, **THE NATURAL HEALER'S ACUPRESSURE HANDBOOK: G-JO FINGERTIP TECHNIQUE**. This technique is a two-step process—first, you must *find the right point*; and, second, you must *stimulate the point properly.* To find the right pressure point, turn to the illustrations on the final pages of this booklet and begin deeply probing that area of your body that corresponds to the illustration. You are looking for a tender "ouch point"—one that feels like a toothache or pinched nerve. You must probe as deeply as you can—up to 20 lbs. of fingertip pressure (use a bathroom scale to see how much 20 lbs. of pressure is)—using the tip (not the pad or fleshy part) of your thumb or the bent knuckle of your index finger if you have long thumbnails. If you are elderly and don't have quite enough strength, use the eraser tip of a pencil (but don't press too deeply, or you might bruise yourself).

Stimulate deeply enough for the point to be quite sensitive, using a digging, goading kind of fingertip massage, for up to four minutes on either side of your body (most of these points are duplicated bilaterally—on either side of the body, that is). These points may be stimulated four or five times a day, symptomatically, on a regular basis. However, acupressure should be avoided *if you are a chronic heart patient—especially if you wear a pacemaker or other artificial energy-regulating device—or if you are a pregnant woman (especially beyond your third month of pregnancy*—however, there are a number of G-Jo acupressure points to aid delivery and recovery if you are having a natural, drugless childbirth).

Acupressure should be used as supportive therapy with other self-health techniques—especially the avoidance of known triggering foods or your own allergens. There are no individual points for *all* forms of arthritis (the following pressure points are mainly pain control points for general use), but many of the points will be beneficial on a broad-spectrum basis. There are numerous other acupressure points for specific bodily areas covered in **THE NATURAL HEALER'S ACUPRESSURE HANDBOOK** that cannot be covered in this booklet because of space restrictions (since you have read this program, you may disregard the suggestion to avoid the use of G-Jo acupressure techniques that is carried in the handbook).

There are several other times when the use of these points should be temporarily avoided—within four hours of taking drugs, medications, alcohol or other intoxicants (acupressure and medications do not mix well, which is generally true of most forms of natural therapy—either use medicines or natural therapy, but do not use both unless suggested/approved by your doctor). . .within half an hour after taking a hot bath, eating a heavy meal or doing physical exercise . . . and if any of the suggested points lie beneath a scar, mole, wart or other blemish, avoid them. Use a different point, instead.

This concludes The G-Jo Institute Arthritis Self-Health Program. We wish you the best of luck and health and offer you our sincere encouragement in your quest for well-being. Any disease can be cured—all it takes is the desire and the continuing effort to become well and healed. Even if it takes longer than you had hoped, have faith. These techniques will work for you, just as they have worked for thousands of other sufferers throughout history. And besides—what better thing do you have to do with your life than to heal yourself?

The G-Jo Institute
Post Office Box 8060,
Hollywood, Florida 33024

SOME USEFUL G-JO ACUPRESSURE POINTS FOR ARTHRITIS SUFFERERS . . .

G-Jo Point No. 115

Midway between the nose and the upper lip.

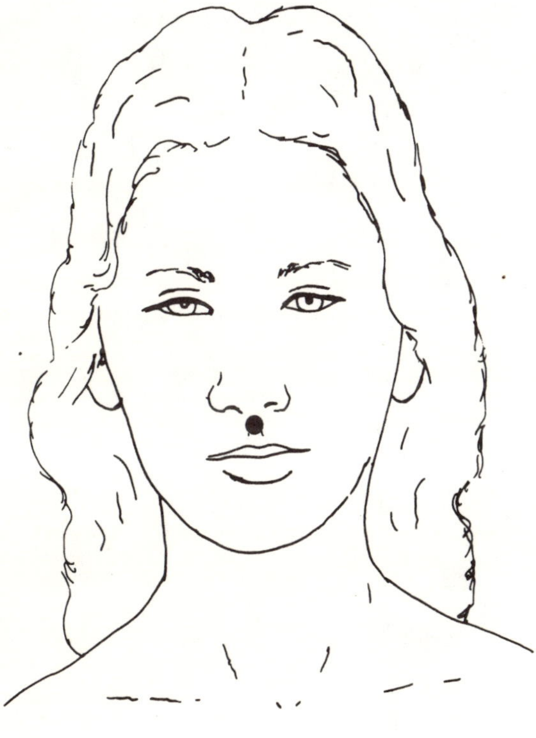

G-Jo Point No. 5

In the hollow (or valley) behind the crown of the *outer* ankle.

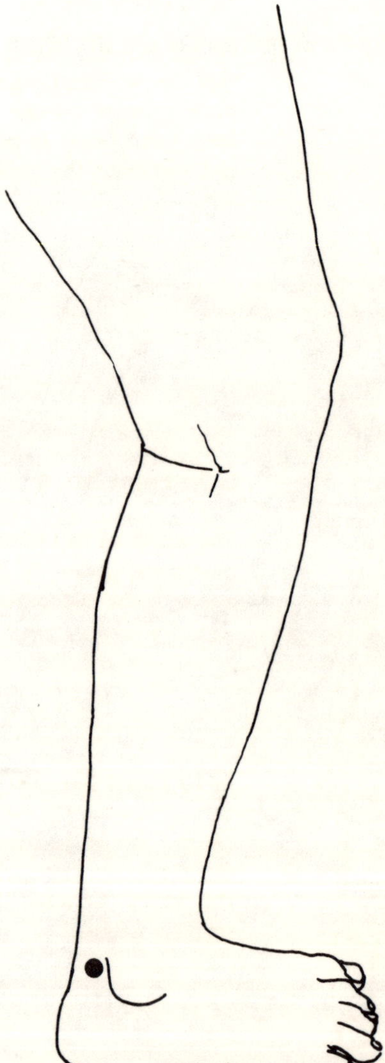

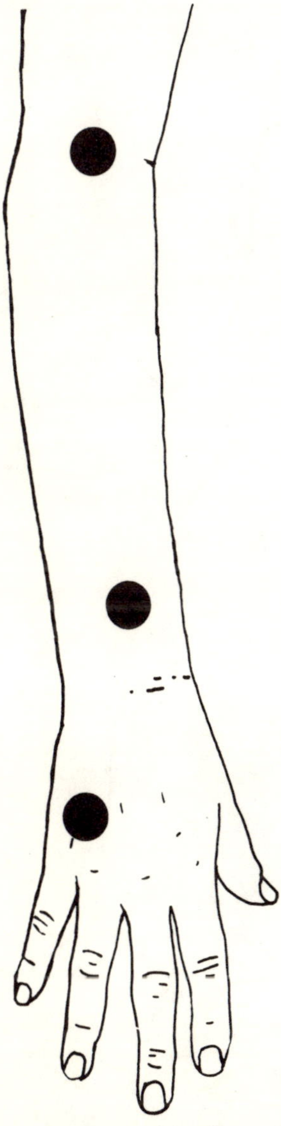

G-Jo Point No. 2

On the extreme end of the outer crease of the elbow. Bend your arm tightly and place a finger on the end of the crease; keep your finger in place. Open the arm and stimulate the point on your relaxed arm.

G-Jo Point No. 4

The width of two thumbs above the most prominent crease of the *upper* wrist, in line with the middle finger.

G-Jo Point No. 38

On the top of the hand, midway between the rearmost knuckles and the wrist; in the valley between the third and the smallest fingers.

G-Jo Point No. 27

The width of two thumbs above the top of the kneecap, in the inner thigh, approximately in line with the crown of the inner ankle.

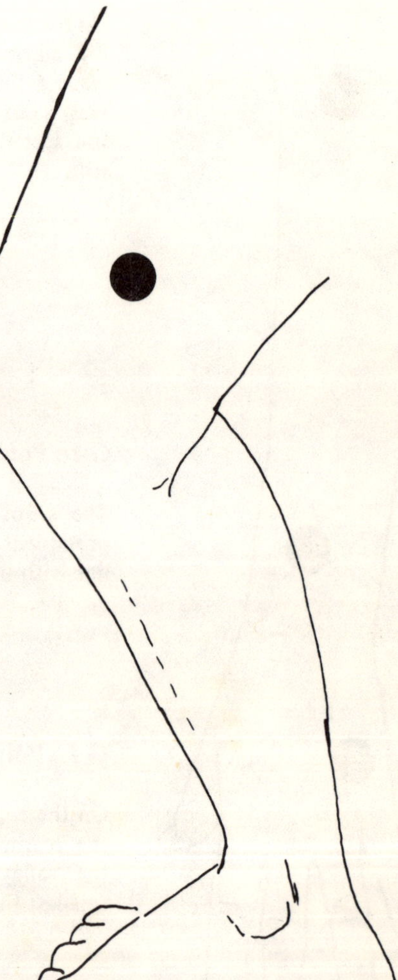